Mental Health? A Mystery.
Mental Illness? Another Mystery.
Your 11th Psychiatric Consultation.
William Yee M.D., J.D.
Copyright Applied for 05/28/2020

First Encounters
1947
I was born in 1947 when my parents lived
on Chene Street, in Detroit Michigan.
I have no memories of that time.

My mother told me that a neighbor
slapped me, and my father got into a fight
with the neighbor. She did not say if it
was a verbal, or a physical fight and I did
not ask.

As a child, I usually listened, and did not
ask many questions.

1950-1953
I lived on a farm near Daggett, Michigan
with my grandparents, an uncle and two
aunts.

My parents lived and worked in Detroit,
Michigan, in restaurants and laundries.

My grandfather worked in a factory in Iron Mountain, Michigan. He visited the farm from time to time.

I became familiar with cows, and milking cows, chickens, and collecting eggs, pastures, cow pies and snow.

I don't recall any sickness during that time of my life.

1953-1958
I lived in the Shady Lane Trailer Park on Capital Street by Nine Mile and Ryan in Warren, Michigan. This was a suburb of Detroit.

My mother came from Daggett, Michigan to Detroit, looking for work.
My father came from China in 1938 to Salt Lake City to work in his father's restaurant when he was fifteen.
He then moved to Detroit, where he met my mother.

Many of my neighbors were migrants from the South who came to Detroit to work in the automobile factories.

It was about 1953 and I was six years old.

The trailers were arranged in two rows with a narrow lane every two rows. The lane was wide enough to drive through, but not wide enough for parking.

The cars were parked outside of the trailers at the edges of the trailer park.

I had a neighbor who lived across the lane. He was slim, about five foot eight, in his forties and soft spoken.

He had large whitish-pink marks on each temple. They were round and about the size of a silver dollar. They stood out on his tanned face. When we talked, he would scratch these spots from time to time.

He noticed me looking at them when he scratched. He was self-conscious about the spots.

He felt compelled to explain it to me. "It's a nervous habit. I can't stop doing it. I have bad nerves."

During the winter, my friend Steven and I asked him if we could shovel the snow off his patio and sidewalk.

We offered to do it for fifty cents.

The snow was wet and so heavy we couldn't do it.

He shoveled the snow and gave us the fifty cents.

I liked him.

It is easy for me to like people, even when they don't give me fifty cents.

Steven's father told me he was a tool and die maker. He said that he went to Brazil to build a factory. He said he was only a tool and die maker, but he was doing the work of an engineer.

Steven's father was drinking milk. He said he put scotch into the milk.

I asked him why he put the scotch into the milk.

Steven's father said that he was an alcoholic, and he drank too much.

He had an ulcer, so he put scotch in milk to make it easier on his ulcer.

I never saw Steven's father drunk. He was always nice to me.

I attended Neigebaur Elementary School, 23068 Ryan Rd, Warren, Michigan from1953 to 1958.

During lunch hour, the school allowed the mentally retarded children out into the playground with the rest of the students.

There was one mentally retarded student who was twice as big as me.

I was small and the only Chinese student on the playground.

I caught his attention. He was mean to me. This made me afraid of mentally retarded students and I avoided them as much as possible.

My father took me to the Hazel Park Raceway, located in Hazel Park, Michigan.

When we were walking into the racetrack, I saw a man with a pregnant woman walking out of the park.

She was crying, "we lost all of our money, it wouldn't have been so bad but....."

Roger took us to a small trailer where a lady lived. She was young. She had very pale skin.

She was soft spoken and very nice.
She told us she had leukemia.
I didn't know what leukemia was.
She didn't look sick, but I understood that it was a serious illness.

She said it made her very tired.
She told us to get some snow.
Roger said, "don't get the yellow snow," and laughed.
When we brought the snow back to her, she mixed it with eggs, sugar, and milk and it was like ice cream.

We visited her only a few times. She was very nice. I liked her a lot. I thought that she was beautiful.

She talked about reading her Bible and the comfort of her religion.

It wasn't long before her small trailer disappeared. I never saw her after that.

I think about her now and then. I miss her when I think about her.

1958
I spent the day at the Cathey House in Lincoln Park, Michigan. My father worked there.

A customer ordered black coffee and burnt toast. He was very thin.
Burnt toast was interesting, I asked,

"Why did you order burnt toast?"
He looked at me, smiled and said,
"I have an ulcer. It helps with the ulcer."
Steven Smith's father had an ulcer and put milk in his scotch. This very thin man had an ulcer and ate burnt toast.

We did not have much to say to each other. He was quiet and polite and easy to like.

A lot to think about.

1958 to 1965
I moved to East Detroit and attended Pleasant View Elementary School, Grant Junior High School and East Detroit High School.

In Junior High School, I met Dennis Cirillo. We both played the saxophone in band class with Mr. Blair.

Dennis Cirillo had a neighbor, John Watkins.
John Watkins had a friend Richard. We visited him at his house a few times.

Richard was very pale and thin. He had leukemia.

Richard was too sick to go to school so he would attend by telephone. Richard would listen to the class and talk on a speaker.

John Watkins visited Richard in the hospital near the end.
He said Richard was so thin it made him sick at heart to see him. Richard had tubes attached to his body to keep him alive and was very weak. He could hardly talk.

John said Richard was his good friend and it was hard to bear.

I felt sorry for them.

I thought about the beautiful lady in the trailer court and how pale she was and how her small green trailer was missing one day. It was all very sad.

1960
In 1960, Thomas Szasz published The Myth of Mental Illness.
Thomas Szasz pointed out that mental illness was without a demonstrated basis in biological science. He pointed out the pressures of politics and economics that created a, "legal fiction," a myth that robbed people of their civil liberties and constitutional rights.

1965-1968
I attended Michigan State University
1965-1966.

I caught the measles and spent the week
sleeping in the campus infirmary to
isolate me from the women on campus
who might be pregnant.

Rubella, also called German measles,
causes birth defects that include deafness,
heart problems, microcephaly, vision
problems, hearing problems, intellectual
disability, bone problems, growth
problems, and liver and spleen damage.

1966-1968
I attended Wayne State University.
I did not meet anyone with medical
problems.
Everyone was working and going to
school.
Wayne students did not party, they
worked.

1967-1971
I was working at the Elden Avenue Gear
and Axel Plant from 1968 to 1971.

I worked the second shift. The second shift was different.

I encountered Gay and Transgender men in the plant.

They found out I was a medical student and they liked to talk to me about gender change surgery.

I liked talking to them.

I was only a medical student and didn't know much. In that respect, I disappointed them.

I met them again in 1973 at a Bette Midler concert, at the Masonic Temple in Detroit.

This was Bette's first national tour. My brother Bob bought the tickets.
I attended the concert with my best friend Vic, his first wife, my brother Bob and his first wife, and my first wife.

I was totally unprepared for the show. We were straight and everyone else in the crowd was in full drag.

They were gays and transgenders.

I recognized some of them from the Eldon Avenue Gear and Axel plant.

The gays and transgenders stared and commented on the "straights," lost in their crowd.

It was an extraordinary concert and an extraordinary evening.

Bette played off the crowd and they played off her as part of the act.

Bette got her start in the bath houses in New York and this was her world. She was theirs.

At that time homosexuality was treated as a mental illness and prosecuted as a crime.

1967
James Riddle Hoffa was imprisoned in 1967 for jury tampering, attempted bribery, conspiracy, and mail and wire fraud.

1968-1972
I attended medical school at Wayne State University from 1968 to 1972.

1969
Ronald L. Krome, M.D. graduated from the Wayne State Surgery residency in 1969.

In 1969 and was put in charge of the Detroit General Hospital emergency room.
The American College of Emergency Physicians (ACEP) was incorporated in 1969.

The American College of Emergency Physicians had its national headquarters in Lansing, Michigan.

Dr. Krome was the editor-in chief of The Annals of Emergency Medicine from 1972-1988.

As a medical student I spent time in the Detroit General Hospital Emergency Room.

There were many mentally ill patients in the Detroit General Hospital Emergency Room.

They were treated for their medical conditions, then, they were transferred to Northville State Hospital.

In medical school I learned that scratching your head until you had round pink spots was a, "tic," and a mental illness.

I learned that drinking too much was alcoholism and a mental illness.

I learned that homosexuality was a mental illness.

I learned that gambling was a mental illness.

I learned that mental retardation was a mental illness.

I thought about my neighbor scratching his head.

I thought about Steven's father drinking scotch in milk.

I thought about the pregnant lady crying at the racetrack.

I thought about the gays and transgenders at the Eldon Avenue Gear and Axle Plant in Detroit, Michigan.

I felt sorry for the crying pregnant lady.

When I talked to the rest of them, they seemed normal to me.

They were nice to me, except for the retarded boy who bullied me on the playground. I didn't like him. I was afraid of him.

I took a three-month rotation in internal medicine.

The resident in training was our proctor. He told us that he had Acanthosis Nigricans. He said that he had a 50% chance of developing cancer.

He did not appear to be physically or mentally ill. He said it matter of factly, calmly, without any drama or apparent distress, stoically.

1972-1975 My Clinical Experience Begins.

I was a resident training in psychiatry at Lafayette Clinic 1972-1973.

Dr. Ralph Slovenko was a professor of law and psychiatry at Wayne State University since 1969.

He received the Manfred Guttmacher Award of the American Psychiatric Association for his book "Psychiatry and Law," published in 1973.

I read The Myth of Mental Illness by Thomas Szasz and some of his other writings.

On the one hand I was required to use the DSM-III. I

I also understood that I was a doctor, a scientist and subject to political and economic forces that undermined the scientific method in medicine.

In 1973 Dr. Ralph Slovenko and Dr. Elliott Luby were interested in finding an effective treatment for the violently mentally ill.

The violently mentally ill were and are notoriously refractory to treatment.

Dr. Ralph Slovenko and Dr. Elliott Luby proposed experimental brain surgery despite the catastrophic history of the lobotomy.

Gabe Kaimowitz, a Michigan Legal Services lawyer, filed a complaint for a Writ of Habeas Corpus on behalf of a "John Doe," Mr. Lois Smith, to stop the experimental surgery.

The result was that medical experiments on prisoners and involuntary psychiatric patients ended abruptly across the country.

It was determined that if you were an involuntary patient, you had no legal capacity to consent to medical experimentation.

I learned that the law, lawyers, and courts had a lot of influence on the practice of medicine and psychiatry.

I trained at Northville State Hospital 1973 to 1975.

I learned that homosexuality was no longer a mental illness.

I learned that the diagnosis of mental illness was based on the DSM-III and that the American Psychiatric Association owned the copyright to the DSM-III.

This was my introduction to the separation of Mental Illness from the Scientific Method.
This was my introduction to the Business of Psychiatry, and the Business of Medicine.

I learned about factitious disorder.

Some patients have a mental illness that involves the need to be mentally or physically ill.

They will fake physical and mental illness They will go from doctor to doctor until they have a diagnosis of physical or mental illness.'

This is called Munchhausen Disorder.

If the parents have a need for their child to be physically or mentally ill, they will take their child from doctor to doctor until they find a doctor that diagnosis a mental illness.

This is called Munchhausen by Proxy.

Sometimes Child Protective Services places the child into foster care to protect the child from their parents and doctors.

That is an interesting thought. Placing a child into Foster Care to protect the child from doctors.

Sometimes the patient will fake a mental illness to get disability income or to sue for a slip and fall or for an injury on the job.

This is called malingering.

It can be very difficult to separate factitious disorder, Munchhausen Disorder and malingering from actual physical and mental illness.

During my residency training we were taught to employ drug free holidays for our psychiatric patients that were on antipsychotic medications like Haldol.

The reason was that the psychiatric literature at that time reported about half the patients in state hospitals developed Tardive Dyskinesia after several years on antipsychotic medications.

Tardive Dyskinesia is the presence of abnormal motor movements at rest. The patient is not able to sit still because of neurological damage to the brain caused by antipsychotic medications.

Part of the reason for the Tardive Dyskinesia was that patients in state hospitals tended to be violent. If they were psychotic and not violent, they were treated in outpatient clinics, not hospitals.

Patients in state hospitals tended to be chronically violent and there were no places other than the state hospital where they could be safely managed.

Patients in state hospitals tend not to respond well to antipsychotic medications so they tend to be on high doses of antipsychotic medications in efforts to overcome the psychosis and violence with the antipsychotic medications.

High doses of antipsychotic medications increase the risk of tardive dyskinesia.

Another reason for drug free holidays is to find out which patients have Tardive Dyskinesia.
Antipsychotic medications mask Tardive Dyskinesia while causing Tardive Dyskinesia.

When the patient tapers off of the antipsychotic medication the Tardive Dyskinesia is unmasked and appears for diagnosis.

Patients will sometimes miss some of their antipsychotic medications, and when the symptoms of Tardive Dyskinesia appear, they will think the symptoms are symptoms of their mental illness getting worse.

When they take their medications, and the Tardive Dyskinesia is masked they think that they are getting better.

In reality, the motor movements of Tardive Dyskinesia are being again masked as the antipsychotic medication continues to increase the brain damage and the severity of the Tardive Dyskinesia.

The end stage of Tardive Dyskinesia is tracheotomies and gastrotomies.

When the Tardive Dyskinesia is severe, it interferes with breathing and swallowing.

The patients have tracheotomies to allow them to breathe.

They cannot swallow food properly and it goes into their lungs.

They have gastrotomies so that they can be fed by tubes directly into their stomachs.

When Tardive Dyskinesia is severe it can appear as constant and grotesque motor movements.

Some patients find Tardive Dyskinesia so cosmetically disfiguring that they will commit suicide.
Sometimes the treatment is worse than the mental illness.

In the 1980's, state hospitals were paying million-dollar judgments for cases of Tardive Dyskinesia.

In the 1980's the cost of paying for judgments for Tardive Dyskinesia and the cost of treating AIDS patients motivated most states to start closing down their state hospitals.

The end game was migration of the mentally ill into jails and prisons because of their violence.

The remaining state psychiatric hospitals tend to be forensic psychiatric hospitals for the incompetent to stand trial and the not guilty by reason of insanity.
1973-1974

While I was at Northville State Hospital, I met residents in training who were moonlighting on the weekends at Detroit General Hospital Emergency Room for extra money.

They told me that all I had to do was go to the Emergency Room and talk to Dr. Krome to get a job.

I met Dr. Krome and we talked. He said he would pay me $16 and hour to work in the emergency room from 9:00 pm Friday night to 7:00 am Saturday morning or from 9:00 pm Saturday night to 7:00 am Sunday morning.

This was a lot more than the three dollars an hour I had been paid to work in the Chrysler automobile factories in Detroit.

I started working in the Detroit General Hospital Emergency Room on weekend nights for Dr. Krome.

One night I saw one hundred patients in the emergency room.

I treated a patient who was foaming at the mouth with fasciculations of the muscles from swallowing malathion insecticide.

A doctor from India told me that this was a common poisoning in India and to give her IV atropine.

I gave her 1mg of atropine i.v. every few minutes until the foaming at the mouth stopped and fasciculations stopped. The total was fifteen to twenty milligrams of atropine.

She woke up and cursed me out for saving her life.

She wanted to be dead and she had not given me permission to save her life.

Another lady came in for treatment of a heart attack. Her husband was at her side and very worried.

I tore her panty hose at the ankles for quick application of the EKG electrodes. She sat up and cursed me like a sailor. She demanded to be discharged immediately.

Apparently, her, "heart attack," occurred during a domestic quarrel.

I cured her heart attack by tearing her panty hose at the ankle.

Many of the patients were mentally ill, and after medical stabilization, were transferred to Northville State Hospital for psychiatric treatment.

In 1974-1975 I did a rotation in neurology at Sinai Hospital as part of my residency training.

During that neurology rotation, I met a patient with Dystonia Musculorum Deformans (DMD). It is also called torsion dystonia. This is a rare, generalized dystonia.

The muscles don't relax, they pull constantly so that the bones become bent and deformed.

Dystonia Musculorum Deformans usually begins in childhood and becomes progressively worse.

Dystonia Musculorum Deformans is caused by a recessive gene so that both parents must transmit the disease to the child.

First cousins are more likely to have the same recessive genes and pass these kinds of diseases to their children.

She was intelligent and knew that she would probably not have had the disease if her parents were not first cousins.

She was very angry at her parents because her parents were first cousins and she inherited her disease from her parents.

She was beautiful, but her body was a twisted cage, a prison that she could not escape. Her muscles were all very tight, painful and had bent her bones.

She could talk, but she could not use her arms, legs or hands. They were all deformed and useless. She talked about the constant pain, the frustration of having a body that was a prison.

She vented her anger at her parents.

She was physically and mentally ill and suffering on both counts.

There was little I could do but allow her to vent her anger.

It was painful to see and it was painful to hear.

That was part of the curse of her life. What she had to say was painful for others to listen to.

That was a long time ago.

She died a long time ago and has escaped her prison of physical and mental pain.

I often felt I could do little for my patients.

Another patient had myesthenia gravis.

I talked to the patient and because of the vigor with which she asserted that she was having an acute attack I diagnosed factitious disorder.

A neurology resident dropped in while I was examining the patient and challenged my diagnosis.

I prepared a butterfly intravenous line, and I attached a syringe with 10 mg of

Tensilon (edrophonium) to the butterfly
line.

Instead of injecting the Tensilon, I pulled
back on the plunger of the hypodermic
needle, and watched the blood flow into
the butterfly intravenous line.

I asked the patient if she was feeling
better. She said she was.

I drew more blood and asked again if she
was feeling better.
The patient again said she was feeling
better. I drew more blood into the line
and asked a third time of the patient was
better.

Again, she said, "yes," she was feeling
better.

I drew the butterfly needle out of the
patient's vein and looked at the neurology
resident.
She turned red. She was angry and
walked away without saying anything.

I had applied the scientific method to ascertain whether the patient was or was not suffering from a myesthenic crises.

She was not.

I did not see any reason for anger. For me it was just being rational and dispassionate, like an Asperger usually is. I don't, however, claim to be Asperger.

1975-1977
James Riddle Hoffa (born February 14, 1913; disappeared July 30, 1975.

I worked at Henry Ford Hospital in Detroit from 1975 to 1977.

There were over 800 consultations with the medical surgical services each year. The first year Dr. Bresnahan and Dr. Pope and I did every third consultation each.

The second year Dr. Bresnahan resigned and I did every other psychiatric consultation with the medical and surgical services with Dr. Pope doing the rest.

I met patients dying of cancer. I would receive a consultation with each of their admissions and assist them with the grief of their mental illness and dying.

I listened and offered what little comfort I could.

I often ordered Brompton's Mixture for their pain.

My recipe for Brompton's Mixture included Morphine, Cocaine, Thorazine, Elavil, and Methamphetamine.

The patients were grateful for the relief from pain and the methamphetamine allowed them to be awake and alert to say their fare wells to their friends and relatives.

I received consultations from the high-risk pregnancy clinic.

One of the patients was fifteen years old. She had been released from the Hawthorn Center. 18471 Haggerty Road. Northville, Michigan 48167.

She was in her second trimester and she was on Mellaril, 400mg three times a day.

I explained the risks and benefits of the medication to the fetus.

She was very concerned about the baby and she wanted to be a good mother.

I found it difficult to see any mental illness during this discussion of the baby's welfare.

I suggested that we taper the medications.

I suggested that we start by reducing the 400mg of Mellaril three times a day to 300mg three times a day for a week, then 200mg three times a day for a week then 100mg three times a day for a week and then stop the Mellaril altogether.

She came back the next week and I asked her how she was doing on three hundred milligrams three times a day.

She was very excited, she said that she had stopped the medications completely and that after she stopped the medications the baby started moving.

She said she had no symptoms of mental illness.

She displayed no symptoms of mental illness and she had no problems during the rest of the pregnancy.

She took the initiative and stopped the medications completely with no catastrophic relapse into mental illness.

Over the years I have had many patients stop their psychotropic medications abruptly without serious adverse effects.

There was no apparent harm to the baby reported from the high-risk pregnancy clinic.

Her judgment was better than mine in that situation.
Stopping the Mellaril abruptly had a better outcome than tapering the medication.

I never saw her after the baby was born.

During our entire time together, I never saw any signs or symptoms of mental illness.

She was a fifteen-year old pregnant girl acting exactly like a responsible parent to be.

She did not use drugs. She did not use alcohol. She did not smoke. She did not use foul language.

She was polite, displayed respect, and proper etiquette at all times.

The medical mystery for me was, "what was she like at the time the Mellaril was raised to 400mg three times a day?"

Perhaps she shall read this book and send me a post card with the rest if her story.

Better yet, maybe she will write her autobiography and give me the opportunity to see myself through her eyes.

1977-1984
I was in private practice from 1977 to 1984

During this period, I found out that I
could treat members of the Teamster's
Union, but their insurance never paid me
for services that I rendered.

During that period, I saw many patients
in consultation at Heritage Hospital in
Taylor Michigan and Outer Drive Hospital
in Lincoln Park, Michigan.

The intensive care unit at Outer Drive
Hospital presented me with three very
difficult cases.

One case was a suicide attempt by
overdose of Elavil.

This case was challenging because the
managed care company wanted me to ask
a severely depressed and suicidal patient
to drive to a psychiatric hospital.
I refused, I ordered and ambulance
transfer because the patient was not safe
outside of constant supervision.

The medical insurance company had the last word.

When I submitted my bill for the psychiatric consultation, they refused to pay.

They asserted that the overdose of Elavil was substance abuse and substance abuse was not covered by the medical insurance policy.

No good deed goes unpunished? Kill the messenger?

Another case was a patient who overdosed on PCP.

PCP is notorious for causing violent psychosis. This patient was in restraints because he was so psychotic and violent.

I ordered Vitamin C to lower the pH of the urine and acidify the urine and remove the PCP faster, a thousand times faster.

The nephrologist ordered the opposite, something to raise the PH and alkalinize the urine to prevent precipitation of myoglobin in the kidneys and to prevent kidney failure.

The result was that this patient took six weeks to get rid of the PCP and the violent psychosis.

This patient remained in physical restraints for six weeks, but he awoke with his kidneys intact and no permanent physical or mental damage from the PCP psychosis.

The third patient in the Outer Drive Intensive Care Unit had ingested Drano as a suicide attempt.

Drano is an alkali that causes rapid liquefaction necrosis to the esophagus.

This results in a fistula between the esophagus and the lungs.

The fistula allows stomach acids to flow into the lungs and results in death.

This is a very slow and painful death that takes about two weeks.

This patient was extremely angry. He refused psychiatric evaluation and treatment.

The attending asked if I could admit him to a psychiatric unit.

I advised the attending that this patient was dying.

I advised the attending that the psychiatric unit did not have the equipment necessary to manage his medical condition.

In addition, I could not admit the patient because he was refusing psychiatric evaluation and treatment.

I came in daily and watched him die. He was in a rage the entire time. He was in pain the entire time.

His death was his wish and his blessing at the end.

I could not offer him anything that he wanted.

He refused treatment because all he wanted was to die and to be free of his anger.

He got his wish.

I was consulted to manage DT's, Delirium Tremens in an alcoholic.

I was treating a lot of alcoholics at that time.

Michigan did not allow the sale of alcohol on Sundays.

Alcoholics would buy Sterno and drink it on Sundays.

Sterno had methanol added to the ethanol so that it could not be sold for human consumption and taxed as an alcoholic beverage.

A can of Sterno could burn for two hours and was used in the catering business to heat food for weddings and other parties.

Alcoholics would buy Sterno on Sunday's because it was cheap and they did not want to go into DT's, Delirium Tremens.

DT's is a painful withdrawal from alcohol that includes psychosis and seizures and can be fatal.

Alcoholics risked methanol poisoning.

Small amounts of methanol, as found in Sterno, have resulted in death. Chronic exposure can cause blindness and kidney failure.

Methanol intoxication and poisoning is where the phrase, "blind drunk," comes from.

I was asked to consult and manage DT's in an alcoholic on the medical unit of Outer Drive Hospital.
I gave the man five milligrams of Valium and it did not touch his delirium. DT's is caused by the lack of alcohol in the brain cells.

The brain cells need either glucose or alcohol for energy.

Alcoholics often get all their calories from alcohol because they often spend all their money on alcohol and nothing on food.

As a result, they do not have thiamine in their brains.

Thiamine is necessary for the metabolism of glucose by brain cells.

This man was in Delirium Tremens. He had no alcohol. He was given food and had sugar, but no thiamine in his brain.

His brain cells were dying as we talked for lack of energy.

I could see the Delirium of Delirium Tremens and knew that his brain cells were dying and that was why he was in delirium.

I ordered an ounce of whiskey.

Within minutes of drinking that ounce of whiskey his delirium cleared up and we had a rational conversation.

I ordered an injection of 100mg of thiamine intramuscularly.

I ordered an ounce of whiskey an hour to keep his brain alive until the thiamine could find its way from his muscle to his brain.

The next day the man remained free of delirium and I stopped the alcohol.

He did not relapse into delirium. I knew that the thiamine was in his brain and his brain was now able to metabolize the sugar for energy.

The man left the hospital with his brain intact. This is one of the few times that I was sure that I had made a difference in a patient's life.
In psychiatry, you treat patients, but you usually have no way of knowing that you made a positive difference with your treatments.

1979-1983

I attended law school. I saw the world differently after going to law school.

I learned about Jimmy Hoffa and the Teamster's Health and Welfare Fund and the Mafia and why I was never paid when I treated these union members for mental illness.

I learned that malingering to obtain disability and medical benefits was a felony and prison time could be substantial.

I learned about taxes, and civil procedure and criminal procedure.

Law school required students to take classes with a written thesis instead of an examination for a grade.

The thinking was that lawyers should be able to write.

This book may demonstrate either failure or success on the part of the law school.

I took two classes in 1983 that required written papers for a grade.

In the first class I wrote a theses title: "Handicap and Access to Medical Care In Hospitals in Michigan, Application of Hospital Rules, By-Laws and Policies," by William R. Yee R. Yee M.D., J.D. Copyright Applied for 1983.

I returned to Lafayette Clinic to take the second class.

Dr. Ralph Slovenko taught a class in Law and Psychiatry at Lafayette Clinic for the Wayne State Universtiy Law School.

I took took Dr. Ralph Slovenko's class. I wrote a paper: "Assault in Hospitals: Theory, Policy and Management." I applied for a copyright for this thesis on Aug 19, 1983.

He gave me an A-. I looked at the A and thought to myself,
"why the minus?"
I did not return to Lafayette Clinic to ask that question.

In law school I learned a lot about contract law and understood how medical insurance policies could alter the practice of medicine.

I also learned about how malpractice insurance could alter the practice of medicine.

I learned that a lot of the people I knew were doing what was considered criminal behavior.

For example, working under the table was tax evasion. It is common among blue collar workers who do not realize how important social security can be during long years of retirement.

1981
March 30, 1981, John Warnock Hinckley Jr. (born May 29, 1955) shot president Ronald Reagan.

John W. Hinckley Jr.'s trial for the shooting of President Reagan was dubbed the war of the experts.

Dr. Park E. Dietz, an assistant professor of psychiatry at Harvard Medical School, helped in the writing of a 628-page report for the prosecution and submitted a bill for $115,917 to the government.

Fourteen doctors took the stand by the eighth week of the trial.

John W. Hinckley Jr's parents were millionaires and spent hundreds of thousands of dollars on lawyers and expert witnesses.

The government spent about a million dollars prosecuting Mr. Hinkley.

The total cost of the lawyers and expert witnesses for the prosecution of Mr. Hinkley is believed to be about another million dollars.

The experts were renowned psychiatrists and neurologists and each side came to the exact opposite conclusion based upon the same facts.

The public's opinion was that you could buy any psychiatric or neurologic opinion you could afford.

This is generalized into the thought that you can find a medical expert to say anything you want to say in court.

The Hinkley trial discredited the science of psychiatry and neurology.

Psychiatry and neurology were reduced to the science of speculation and conjecture outside of the scope of the scientific method.

1987
I started working in prisons.
Since 1987 I have worked at Michigan Dept. of Corrections, 777 W. Riverside Drive Ionia, Michigan 48846 from 1987 to 1991;
Muskegon Correction Facility and E. C. Brooks Correctional Facility from 02/22/08 to 02/13/0;
Bellamy Creek Correctional Facility (IBC) in Ionia Michigan from 06/01/2009 to 03/26/2010;

California State Prison, Sacramento
(SAC) - California 100 Prison Road,
Represa, CA 95671 from 02/07/2011 to
03/13/2012;
Pelican Bay State Prison, (the only
supermax facility in the state of
California), 5905 Lake Earl Dr, Crescent
City, CA 95532 from 04/09/2012 to October
16, 2013;
ICF Ionia Correctional Facility, also
known as "I-Max," once a Level VI
Supermax, now a Level V prison, 1576 W.
Bluewater Highway. Ionia, MI
48846, from November 4, 2013 to January
2, 2015;
San Quentin State Prison (SQ) San
Quentin, CA 94964, from 09-08-2014 to 12-
31-2014
Bellamy Creek Correctional Facility, 1727
Bluewater Hwy, Ionia, MI 48846 from
January 5, 2015 to February 6, 2015;

I learned that Antisocial Personality
Disorder is a mental illness in private
practice, but not in prison.
Prisons are a stressful work environment
and I learned a great deal about stress,
mental health, and mental illness.

Staff in prisons suffer from stress.

1988
In 1988 Stephen William Hawking published a popular book about physics, <u>A Brief History of Time: From the Big Bang to Black Holes</u>.

I found out that in 1963, Hawking was diagnosed with amyotrophic lateral sclerosis or Lou Gehrig's disease.

I thought about the young lady with dystonia musculorum deformans, and how different her life was from the life of Mr. Hawking.

Hawking was trapped in the prison of his body, but his mind was free to explore the universe.

Hawking looked outward and forward.

The lady with dystonia musculorum deformans looked inwards and backwards. She could not get past the anger and grief of having her disease.

Hawking had a normal youth, she did not.

1989
In 1989 Joseph Lyle Menéndez and Erik Galen Menéndez murdered their parents.

1994
In 1994 Joseph Lyle Menéndez and Erik Galen Menéndez were convicted of murdering their parents with shotguns.

Their defense was that they murdered their parents because of years of sexual and emotional abuse.

The jury found them guilty, and apparently thought the brothers were malingering and not mentally ill.
I thought about the Hinkley trial, the war of the experts and how psychiatrists had lost credibility with the general public.
2012

Thomas Stephen Szasz fell and broke the tenth vertebrae of his spine. Less than a week later he committed suicide in his home in Manlius, New York on September 8, 2012.

2013

Ronald L. Krome, MD, FACEP (E), the sixth president of the American College of Emergency Physicians, died May 23., 2013. He was 77. He had many admirers, "A visionary, supreme clinician, scholar and above all just a great person. We all a blessed to have a little of him in us. Because of this, he will live forever. We love you Ron and your wonderful family."

2016

Gainesville attorney Gabe Kaimowitz has been disbarred for continuing to practice law after he was suspended by the Florida Supreme Court in 2014.

2015 to the Present

In 2015 I started working in State Forensic Psychiatric Hospitals.
Atascadero State Hospital, from February 9, 2015 to May 18, 2017.
Patton State Hospital from May 22, 2018 to January 18, 2018.
Kalamazoo Psychiatric Hospital, April 16, 2018 to November 15, 2018.

I learned a lot about mental illness and incompetent to stand trial, not guilty by reason of insanity, and malingering in the criminal justice system.

2016
John W. Hinckley Jr. Is released from a government hospital in 2016.

2016
Dr. Ralph Slovenko, died Nov. 3, 2016 in Detroit. He was 86 and a respected forensic psychologist when he died.

However, some saw fit to post disparaging remarks about him on the internet after his death. He did not have the wide respect that Dr. Krome commanded.

2018
Hazel Park Raceway closed in April, 2018. I think about pregnant lady crying and all the people I had met that had problems in their lives because they could not control their gambling.

2020
I stand before you ready to answer
questions to the best of my ability.

The patient comes to me and wants to
know what is wrong and how to fix it.

"Doctor, what is wrong with me?"

The answer is basically, "I don't know."

The patient asks me, "what is my
diagnosis?

What do I say next?
"Tell me more."

The patient may identify the problems as
emotions, stress, behaviors, thinking.

What do I say next?
"OK, you say your problems are
emotional. The emotions can be
depression, anxiety, anger, grief."
"The science of psychiatry is not able to
pinpoint where in your 100 billion
neurons and 1000 trillion synapses the

depression, anxiety, anger and grief are causing your inability to function effectively."

"Psychiatry has the convention of calling collections of symptoms mental illness."

"For example, the American Psychiatric Association has collections of symptoms with names that are copyrighted in the The Diagnostic and Statistical Manual of Mental Disorders, Fifth Edition (DSM-5)."

"The DSM-5 is a manual for assessment and diagnosis of mental disorders. Each diagnosis is like a recipe in a cookbook."

"Collections of emotional symptoms are called Major Depression or Bipolar Disorder or Mood Disorder Not Otherwise Specified, or Anxiety disorder, or Panic Disorder, or Social Anxiety Disorder or Phobia, etc."

"Psychiatry is in the posture that medicine was before germs were discovered."

"People had pneumonia, with fever and cough and they died but nobody knew anything about germs."

"They talked about vapors and humors and curses and hexes. They could offer aspirin for the fever and cooling baths. That all changed with the discovery of germs."

"Psychiatrists cannot tell the patient that they actually know what the mental illnesses are."

"If you read the package inserts and the FDA Labels for psychiatric medications they say, 'the mechanism of action is not known.'"

"Because the mental illness is not actually known the basis for the improvements with the medications are not actually known."

The patient asks,
"OK, Dr. Yee, you do not know what mental illness is, can you treat it?"

My answer is,
"yes, I can treat it, in the same way that aspirin treats pneumonia. I cannot cure your mental illness, but I can offer a medication that reduces the severity of symptoms for many patients, but not all patients."

"Psychiatry offers antidepressants and antipsychotics for the fevers of mental illness."

The thinking of Thomas Szasz in many ways remains valid. There is still a great deal of politics, economics, and money that moves psychiatry outside of the scope of the scientific method.

Psychiatrists do not have the cures that penicillin and other antibiotics offer.

Let us examine Major Depressive Disorder.

Major Depressive Disorder manifests with depressed mood most of the day almost every day. Depressed mood may be described as sadness, emptiness of emotions, pervasive hopelessness, loss if interest or the ability to enjoy usual activities.

Review of the medical literature results in at least one opinion that antidepressant medications are no better than a placebo.

Please review:
"Considering the methodological limitations in the evidence base of antidepressants for depression: a reanalysis of a network meta-analysis," Klaus Munkholm, Asger Sand Paludan-Müller, and Kim Boesen; BMJ Open. 2019; 9(6): e024886; Published online 2019 Jun 27. doi: 10.1136/bmjopen-2018-024886; PMCID: PMC6597641; PMID: 31248914
Now let us consider antipsychotic medications.

Perphenazine is as effective as olanzapine, quetiapine, risperidone, and ziprasidone.
Perphenazine is the most cost effective medication for the treatment of psychosis.

You can expect three out of four patients to stop antipsychotic medications within eighteen months due to side effects or failure of benefit to justify the time and money to continue the treatments.

See:
"What CATIE Found: Results From the Schizophrenia Trial," Dr. Marvin S. Swartz, M.D., T. Scott Stroup, M.D., M.P.H., Dr. Joseph P. McEvoy, M.D., Dr. Sonia M. Davis, Dr.P.H., Dr. Robert A. Rosenheck, M.D., Dr. Richard S. E. Keefe, Ph.D., Dr. John K. Hsiao, M.D., and Dr. Jeffrey A. Lieberman, M.D.; Psychiatr Serv. 2008 May; 59(5): 500–506.; doi: 10.1176/ps.2008.59.5.500; PMCID: PMC5033643; NIHMSID: NIHMS816833; PMID: 18451005

There are many criticisms of the CATIE trials. See:
"CATIE & You, What happens when drugs are found to be unsafe and ineffective? Not much.," by Ben Hansen, MindFreedom Michigan, Ragged Edge Online Home

Now let us consider antidepressant medications.

Depression may cause substantial change in weight either up or down.

There may be insomnia or hypersomnia.

Depression may cause pseudo-dementia with memory problems due to lack of attention and impaired concentration.

There may be agitation or fatigue.

Depression may cause feelings of worthlessness or guilt without a basis in reality.

There may be preoccupation with death or suicidal thoughts, plans, impulses or attempts.

Let us examine The STAR*D Trial completed in 2006. In that trial 4,041 outpatients were treated with medications and psychotherapy Patients were treated with the selective serotonin reuptake inhibitor (SSRI) citalopram for up to 14 weeks.

The remission rate was 28-33% and the response rate was 47%.

If the patients did not respond to citalopram, there were offered other antidepressants and cognitive behavioral therapy (CBT) which had a remission rate of 30.6%.

If the patients did not respond they were offered lithium or triiodothyronine (a thyroid hormone) to their antidepressant or mirtazapine or venlafaxine.

The remission rates were
12.3% for mirtazapine and
19.8% for nortriptyline.
The remission rates
15.9% for lithium and
24.7% for triiodothyronine.

If they did not respond they were offered tranylcypromine, or a venlafaxine and mirtazapine combination with a remission rate was 13%.

The odds of beating the depression diminish with each treatment offered in this sequence.

Also, each treatment required 3 to 5 weeks to determine a treatment failure.

The adverse effects were experienced before the benefits of the treatments.

The result of the Star Trial is that about 30% of patients who are treated with psychotropic medications do not respond to treatment.

Of those that respond to treatment to medications, there is a substantial relapse rate back into depression

The Star-D report was challenged by Robert Whitaker: The STAR*D Scandal: A New Paper Sums It All Up, Detailing the methods of dishonest science, Posted Aug 27, 2010, Robert Whitaker.

In his article Mr. Whitaker reports that only 3% of patients had a "sustained remission" and stayed in the trial, despite the assertions in the Star-D study that 40% of the patients had a "sustained remission" and stayed in the trial.

Other studies examine the failures of antidepressant as opposed to their successes.

Original Investigation June 5, 2019, "Efficacy of Esketamine Nasal Spray Plus Oral Antidepressant Treatment for Relapse Prevention in Patients With Treatment-Resistant Depression" A Randomized Clinical Trial"
Ella J. Daly, MD1; Madhukar H. Trivedi, MD2; Adam Janik, MD3; et alHonglan Li, MD, PhD1; Yun Zhang, PhD4; Xiang Li, PhD5; Rosanne Lane, MAS6; Pilar Lim, PhD6; Anna R. Duca, BSN1; David Hough, MD1; Michael E. Thase, MD7; John Zajecka, MD8; Andrew Winokur, MD, PhD9,10; Ilona Divacka, MBA, MD11; Andrea Fagiolini, MD12; Wiesław J. Cubała, MD, PhD13; István Bitter, MD, PhD14; Pierre Blier, MD, PhD15; Richard

C. Shelton, MD16; Patricio Molero, MD, PhD17; Husseini Manji, MD1; Wayne C. Drevets, MD3; Jaskaran B. Singh, MD3

JAMA Psychiatry. 2019;76(9):893-903.
doi:10.1001/jamapsychiatry.2019.1189

The authors set the stage for how important their study is. They state that depression is the most serious mental illness worldwide.

The authors claim that depression shortens life by an average of ten years.

The authors also claim that depression is, "the leading cause of disability worldwide."

The authers then claim a 73% stable remission with the use of intranasal Esketamine.

This is a major advance in the treatment of depression.

Johnson & Johnson (JNJ), set a list price of $590 to $885 per treatment session.

Your insurance may or may not pay for Esketamine treatments.

At $590 and $885 per dose, with the usual treatment being two doses a week the cost of Spravato in the first month of treatment ranges from $4,720 to $6,785.

Good luck asking your insurance to pay for this treatment.

In Summary:
You ask, "doctor, what is my diagnosis?"

My answer is,
"The diagnosis of mental illness is simply a collection of symptoms without a true understanding of the mental illness."

"A jury may find that you are not mentally ill and malingering to escape prosecution for a crime or to commit the crime of fraud to obtain a disability income or a judgment for an injury you did not have."

You ask, "can you treat my mental illness?"

I answer:
"Yes, I can treat your mental illness. But the medications are not as effective as the research and the advertising imply or claim. The medications do not cure mental illness. We will probably both be disappointed in the results offered by the medications I can prescribe."

At this point let us change the strategy of diagnosis and treatment.

Instead of focusing on diagnosis that is necessary for insurance payments, let us focus on symptoms.

It is easier to treat symptoms than diagnosis

Anxiety is a symptom. Rate your anxiety on a scale of 0 to 10 with 0 being no anxiety and ten being the worst anxiety you have ever experienced.

We will treat your anxiety with exercise, deep breathing, meditation, and psychotherapy.

If these don't work, we will add medications.

If you insist, I will start medications today.

You will rate your anxiety in a daily diary and on your next visit we will review your diary and adjust your medications.

You will practice good sleep hygiene.

You will go to sleep and get up at the same time every day.

You will limit caffeine to two or three cups of coffee in the morning and no coffee after twelve noon.

You will do aerobic exercise in the morning under the supervision of your primary doctor.

You will use the bed for sleep and not for watching TV or listening to music.

Your bedroom with be dark and quiet when you sleep.

You will use bright lights when you get up to reboot your sleep cycles.

You will drink chamomile tea with lavender and use melatonin at night to improve sleep.

If these do not work you will ask your primary physician for a referral to a sleep clinic for a sleep EEG to identify Narcolepsy, Sleep Apnea and other medical conditions that cause insomnia.

You will rate your insomnia in a daily diary and on your next visit we will review your diary and consider psychotherapy and other interventions for insomnia at your next visit.

We will treat your hallucinations, delusions, and paranoia with exercise, deep breathing, meditation, and psychotherapy. If these don't work, we will add medications.

If you insist, I will start medications today.

You will rate your hallucinations, delusions, and paranoia in a daily diary and on your next visit we will review your diary and adjust your medications.

The above are examples of treating symptoms based upon evidence based practices.

The diary is the evidence used to modify the treatment to your version of mental illness.

Penicillin for pneumonia, Insulin for diabetes and Viagra for impotence are the Gold Standard for treating medical conditions.

When there is a SchizophreniaViagra for schizophrenia, when there is a BipolarViagra for Bipolar Disorder, when there is a SchizoaffectiveViagra for

Schizoaffective disorder psychiatry will have caught up with other branches for medicine.

For now, psychiatrists are like the seven blind men examining the elephant. One feels the tusk, one feels the tail, one feels the trunk, one feels the leg, one feels the ear and one feels the belly.

No psychiatrist sees the whole picture sufficiently to identify the cause and the cure of mental illness.

There are a few examples in psychiatry where the cause is known sufficiently to offer a, "cure."

Systemic Lupus Erythymatois causes an acute encephalopathy which manifests with a delirium that remits with prednisone treatments.

Acute Intermittent Porphyria can manifest with a psychosis that will remit with a single dose of 150mg of chlorpromazine.

Thiamine deficiency manifests with acute delirium that remits with a combination of alcohol and thiamine and glucose in alcoholics.

The alcohol is necessary to preserve neurons while thiamine is absorbed and allows the neurons to resume the use of glucose for neuron functioning.

I will stop writing at this point.

There is much more literature on the diagnosis and treatment of mental illness.

However, writing must stop at some arbitrary point.

I believe that I have written enough to allow the reader to explore the boundaries of the diagnosis and treatment of mental illness as it progresses in the future.

Thank you for your time and attention. William R. Yee, M.D., J.D. Board Certified Psychiatrist, practicing psychiatry without interruption from 1972 to the present in Michigan, Indiana, Kentucky and California and recently licensed in Texas, at your service.

"Preexisting text," includes names of people and corporations, names of law cases, and text of statutes cited, the titles of articles and books and the content of articles and books cited in the materials above.

My copyright claim is a clam to the "original text," which is my personal experiences as described in the text above and my commentary on the people and corporations, law cases, and text of statutes cited, the articles and books and the content of articles and books cited in the text above.

Preexisting Text is:
The Myth of Mental Illness, Thomas Szasz, 1960

"Handicap and Access to Medical Care In Hospitals in Michigan, Application of Hospital Rules, By-Laws and Policies," by William R. Yee R. Yee M.D., J.D. Copyright Applied for 1983.

"Assault in Hospitals: Theory, Policy and Management." I applied for a copyright for this thesis on Aug 19, 1983.

The Diagnostic and Statistical Manual of Mental Disorders, American Psychiatric Association, DSM-III, DSM-V

<u>A Brief History of Time: From the Big Bang to Black Holes,</u> Stephen William Hawking 988

"A visionary, supreme clinician, scholar and above all just a great person. We all a blessed to have a little of him in us. Because of this, he will live forever. We love you Ron and your wonderful family." "the mechanism of action is not known."

"Considering the methodological limitations in the evidence base of antidepressants for depression: a reanalysis of a network meta-analysis," Klaus Munkholm, Asger Sand Paludan-Müller, and Kim Boesen; BMJ Open. 2019; 9(6): e024886; Published online 2019 Jun 27. doi: 10.1136/bmjopen-2018-024886; PMCID: PMC6597641; PMID: 31248914

What CATIE Found: Results From the Schizophrenia Trial," Dr. Marvin S. Swartz, M.D., T. Scott Stroup, M.D., M.P.H., Dr. Joseph P. McEvoy, M.D., Dr. Sonia M. Davis, Dr.P.H., Dr. Robert A. Rosenheck, M.D., Dr. Richard S. E. Keefe, Ph.D., Dr. John K. Hsiao, M.D., and Dr. Jeffrey A. Lieberman, M.D.; Psychiatr Serv. 2008 May; 59(5): 500–506.; doi: 10.1176/ps.2008.59.5.500; PMCID: PMC5033643; NIHMSID: NIHMS816833; PMID: 18451005

"CATIE & You,What happens when drugs are found to be unsafe and ineffective? Not much.," by Ben Hansen, MindFreedom Michigan, Ragged Edge Online Home
The STAR*D Trial
The STAR*D Scandal: A New Paper Sums It All Up, Detailing the methods of

dishonest science, Posted Aug 27, 2010,
Robert Whitaker

Original Investigation June 5, 2019,
"Efficacy of Esketamine Nasal Spray Plus
Oral Antidepressant Treatment for
Relapse Prevention in Patients With
Treatment-Resistant Depression"
A Randomized Clinical Trial"
Ella J. Daly, MD1; Madhukar H. Trivedi,
MD2; Adam Janik, MD3; et alHonglan Li,
MD, PhD1; Yun Zhang, PhD4; Xiang Li,
PhD5; Rosanne Lane, MAS6; Pilar Lim,
PhD6; Anna R. Duca, BSN1; David Hough,
MD1; Michael E. Thase, MD7; John
Zajecka, MD8; Andrew Winokur, MD,
PhD9,10; Ilona Divacka, MBA, MD11;
Andrea Fagiolini, MD12; Wiesław J.
Cubała, MD, PhD13; István Bitter, MD,
PhD14; Pierre Blier, MD, PhD15; Richard
C. Shelton, MD16; Patricio Molero, MD,
PhD17; Husseini Manji, MD1; Wayne C.
Drevets, MD3; Jaskaran B. Singh, MD3;
JAMA Psychiatry. 2019;76(9):893-903.
doi:10.1001/jamapsychiatry.2019.1189

www.ingramcontent.com/pod-product-compliance
Lightning Source LLC
Chambersburg PA
CBHW021901170526
45157CB00005B/1911